I0468467

Target Secrets for Easy Weight Loss

Ten simple steps for success; Real weight loss, for real people in the real world, which really works.

By Dr Phil Harley

International Copyright 2016

Published by BrainSolutions

All rights reserved

target weight loss ways
time to get into action

Get going today
Use today's motivation
Sustained approach
Can use for ever
Not a diet to try and fail at
No yo-yoing

Do you want to be thinner? Do you want a better waistline? Do you want more energy each day and to feel better about your body?

Me too. This book explains just how to do it.

There are other books out there which will tell you about the next craze, the next must-do diet and how celebrities have secrets the rest of us don't yet know. This isn't one of those books. This is better.

This book explains ten easy to follow steps which actually work. Written by doctors, these will help you safely and effectively lose your waistline and keep it off.

Today you feel positive, so use that. Take a step today. Then do another tomorrow. Keeping sustained effort is all about making it easier. No one likes hard work. Certainly no one likes to work hard when they don't need to or if they aren't rewarded for it.

To make anything easier, make it a habit. Habits take between two weeks and two months to groove in our brains, but each day they take less and less effort. That is what we are after here. Daily actions that get easier and easier. Then you can keep up what needs to be done, forever, with minimal effort.

real world doctors
this stuff really works

Specialist weight loss service
Real world medicine
It really works

- What really really works is stuff which is in harmony with your life.
- Stuff you will do day in and day out.
- Stuff you give up on after six months isn't what you are after. This is for ever. You want to your body last for years - well, here is how to do it:

Food modification AND increased exercise.

This works best. I've not had more than a handful of people in all the thousands I've seen, succeed without cranking up their daily activities.

My wife says doing stuff around the house doesn't count and you need to get your butt all sweaty with huffing and puffing, *proper* exercise. Other people say that you can include everything, even getting up to physically change the TV channel (rather than using the remote).

I don't care who you believe. The point is that if you want this to work you will have to crank up activity levels. And you *DO* want it to work don't you? The point is that your efforts on changing what goes in the top end needs to be matched by lots of output. Lots of little things each and every day. Lots of sneaky little bits of exercise. Lots of extra steps, work on your core, work on your posture. Then go and play sport. Hit the gym, get out on the trails at the weekends. Do whatever works for you. But do it. Do it often and don't have too many off days. Five exercise days and two rest days each week will see you hurtle towards your goals.

Plus you get to feel really great too. Win Win.

Sleep is not to be underestimated. Get more sleep. Really. Eight hours a night. We go through this later. But it is so vital that I will hammer the point home. Get more sleep. Sleep better. Sleep longer. You need it. You deserve it and it will make you happier, thinner, live longer, less likely to get cancer **and** enhance your sex life. *Really* win win.

interlinking strands
how it fits together

The vital trio
Body, mind, spirit
Holistic approach

Based on real modern medical evidence. This approach to making the most of your body and getting you the fastest, most effective, sustainable weight loss is based on real world medicine. Science that works. On real people. In the real world.

Whole person medicine. We are all rather complex. We all have complicated lives. And that's ok. What works for my other patients will work for you too. Handily we are all wired the same and have the same cells that are powered by the same biological urges. We understand them and that is why this approach will work for you.

The vital trio (we'll cover all of this):

-Body
Move more
Fuel well
Forget superfoods
More protein
Slow release stuff

-Mind
Be whelmed
Be busy
Learn about hunger

-Spirit

Rest

Recuperation

Have a purpose

Be entertained

Watch for three snack pitfalls:

- Bored
- Comfort
- Absent minded

Address these and everything else will slot into place.

the ten
top ten action chapters

Do the list
Aimed like a laser
Live longer

Ten things to work on. Take one a day. Pick one a week.

Do them in order, do them out of order. The choice is entirely yours. If in doubt, go for one a day and then cycle back to the beginning. Each time around you will have learned more about how to do stuff better. You will find out what works for *you* in *your* life. You will see what needs more attention and what comes more easily to you.

There is no benefit in staying as you are. If you were pleased with the situation you wouldn't be reading this.

The time is nigh, the time is now. Today is the day. Today is your day. Make it yours.

You will need to be single point focused. Make your mission the most important thing you are doing. Do it every day. Keep it constantly at the front of your mind. Talk about it to everyone. Get help, buddy up, blog about it and post to the book of faces. Keep on task. Make this weight loss mission your most important, highest, first priority.

And it *is* the most important thing. Looking after your physical and mental health is *the* most important thing you can do for you, your long life and for your children. Not a bad return on your efforts for only a few simple steps to follow each day.

You will have noticed this is a small book. That is ok. This is deliberate.

"Small is beautiful."
Leopold Kohr (1909 – 1994), economist and political writer.

Being short, this makes it easy to read. Also easy re-read and simple to digest.

one
what is your goal?

Towards goals
Be specific
Give it some pizazz and wow

When I meet patients in my specialist clinic I can tell very quickly the ones who will do well and the ones who will not do so well. I'm usually right. I love to be proved wrong and have people succeed. But sometimes the writing is on the wall.

People who want to lose weight usually don't. I'm not saying they can't or never do, but that goal is too wishy-washy. It is nebulous, it has no zing, pizazz or razzmatazz about it. Goals which drive people forward include; I want to be sexy for my wedding, I want to see my children grow up, I want to run a marathon.

These are **to**-goals not **away**-goals. This means they want something specific. We can aim towards them in a forward direction. Most of us work much better when we are pulled towards something. If we are pushed away from something (I *don't* want my back to hurt, I *don't* want to be laughed at, I *don't* want to feel this way) humans don't tend to do so well. We don't process negatives well. Try not to think of elephants. You have to think of one in order not to think about them, and this gets the focus all wrong. Find a way to state all your goals as something specific you want.

You are going to need a lot of willpower, energy and mental resources if you are going to change your habits. If you are going to change the way you shop, cook, snack, move around each day and sleep, you are going to need a jolly good reason for doing that or it just ain't going to happen.

I don't want for you to try something, get a tiny taste of success, bump up against the inevitable speedbumps which happen in our lives and then give up and go back to square one. I want you to succeed. You want you to succeed. That is only going to happen with daily consistent action and tuning this new healthier you into a way of life you can be proud of, can share with others and can wear, satisfied and happy every day for the rest of your life.

I don't want something which is only going to give a brief result and nor do you. They can all too easily be undone in a lively weekend. This is for the long haul. If it is for the long haul then you are going to be needing to do stuff day-in and day-out for a very long time. It has to fit, it has to be comfortable and be something you feel okay about, feel good about and can keep up the efforts at.

So my friend, you are going to need a motivating goal. *Capiche?* Really motivating. For you. Not my goal (you'd hate them, they are all about boring running), you need the one about you being super-sexy-naked in front of the bathroom mirror - that sort of thing. You don't have to share these goals with other people. I'd love you to email me and tell me about them. And how you're getting on. But you can keep them inside and feel pleased about them if you'd prefer.

Goals shared and particularly those shared on social media get better results. If you set goals out loud, people will hold you to them. You become socially accountable. And other people do love to help. They really do. You'd help someone else in their quest. They in turn will help you. They will ask for nothing in return and feel good about themselves for simply having helped. You would. Why not allow others to help you? This isn't selfish. They will feel good - so why deny them the chance for that? It would be selfish *not* to share you goals.

Write one. Right now. Write now. Don't worry if it's not perfect, you can revise it, rewrite it, completely change it, hone it or tinker with it later. The point is write one down now. On a physical bit of paper. This has a powerful effect on our brains. It really works. I'll wait for you.

Done it? Go on, I'll wait.

Done now? Good - turn the page.

two
monitor weight

Statistical noise
Trends
Use technology
Same scales
Water
Bowels
Fat
Muscle mass

Measuring stuff brings about better results. Measurable results. Tautology aside, the Hawthorne effect in psychology teaches us that if you measure stuff, it gets done better.

You brain is hardwired to pay attention to stuff. If you measure your weight, your brain will be working in the background to help you achieve your goal. Amazing but true.

If you take more measurements, you will iron out statistical noise. If you have two data points this could give you a perfectly accurate trend. Or it might not. If you measure three thousand, you will be more likely to get a true result.

The sweet spot is daily weights. Same you, each day, same scales. At the same time of day. In your undies. On a hard surface. Write them down, plot them on a spreadsheet. Put this chart on your refrigerator.

Your body weight will go up and down throughout the day. That's ok. It is the trend as the weeks go by that matter. Some days you will have more water in your system and more poop in your guts than at other times. That's also ok and perfectly normal. Measure lots of readings and these differences become less important against the trend over time.

One pound of fat weighs the same as a pound of muscle. If you aren't losing weight but look better and your middle is smaller, it may be that you are putting on muscle mass. This is a good thing. Use waist measurements and eyeball yourself (honestly) in the mirror. Some people put on more muscle than they lose fat and are grumpy about weight gain. But this is rare. Most of my patients put on muscle and lose lots more fat, so still lose weight while becoming healthier and a better shape.

I'm always a bit suspicious of patients who tell me they are still gaining weight with the strategies I give them. Usually they've done something wrong. Most commonly they aren't burning as many calories through exercise as they think or their portion sizes are still too large.

three
count intake

Hawthorne
Daily detail
Calories

This Hawthorne effect and its benefits extend to your daily calorie intake. It's simple: measure what goes in. Day after day you will do better. Though you will need to be brutally honest about what goes in the top end. Really truthful. The biggest errors are in portion sizes and drinks. People forget that most drinks contain calories and these get underestimated. Portion sizes in real life are at least 50% bigger than those on packets. My patients also underestimate calories in butter / spread / oils and fats used in cooking and on bread.

If in doubt, drop the bread and cook without fat - or buy a one-calorie per squirt spray.

Measure everything that goes in. Do this every day until you get really good at judging. Most of us need about a month or two to get the hang of this as it is more tricky than we imagine.

Get in the habit of checking every label, write it all down. Write down the weights of every foody thing you eat.

Prepare stuff yourself and you will know it has no hidden calories. It is also much much better for you. Food prepared by you has much more in the way of protein, vitamins and fiber. Longer and healthier lives await those who chop and prepare their own vegetables.

four
portion size

Plate size
Learn to leave
20, 20, 20

If you eat big portions you will wear bigger pants. Smaller portions and you get to wear smaller pants. That is the deal.

If you fill a big plate, you will naturally want to eat it all. You may or may not feel hungry at the end. If you fill a smaller plate you will be just as likely to feel hungry afterwards as this emotional signal is mainly in your head - but you will have eaten a lot less.

It sounds bats-crazy but it's true. Try it out.

And you will eat a lot less food. A 30cm plate has a surface area of $707cm^2$. A 20cm plate has a surface area of $314cm^2$. That's right, a slightly smaller diameter plate - *only a bit and you could probably make that adjustment* - has less than half the surface area of the bigger plate.

And that's if you cram food to the edge. If you compare food spread to a 1cm margin on the bigger plate and are able to leave a two centimeter margin on the smaller plate, this works out as $615cm^2$ down to $254cm^2$ (a 59% reduction).

It's all about having a **slightly smaller** plate and filling it **slightly less**. You will reap the **huge benefits**.

We are taught as children to finish up our plates. That's ok, but you aren't a child anymore and you are no longer child size. Possibly the size of someone who has eaten a small child, so new rules apply: **Learn to leave a morsel.** This will take some doing at first but gives you a sense of wellbeing and self-control.

It is the human advanced part of your brain giving the basic animal part the message that it is full.

20,20,20 is a strategy which works better for some patients than others. Try it out for a week or two and see if you are one of the hyper-responders.

Each forkful should be the size of a **twenty** pence piece, chewed **twenty** times and each meal should last you **twenty** minutes. This limits the size of your mouthful (a 20p is the same diameter as a US Nickel = 21.4mm). The food is allowed to savor in the mouth, which increases the sensory food experience. Many people find this revolutionizes their experience of eating. They are forced (by these admittedly completely artificial rules) to take time over their food. A full twenty minutes of sit-down time with each meal.

Try it today. You may be pleasantly surprised.

five
swaps for better choices

Low calorie
Less fat, more protein
Slower release energy

Food swaps are trendy and many websites can be found offering their advice and tips on what to eat and what not to eat.

I don't really care too much what you eat. Humans evolved as omnivores, we were hunter-gatherers and thrived. We became farmers and thrived. Now in an industrial setting we thrive. And whatever happens next, we will probably thrive then too. We are at our healthiest when we eat a wide range of foods. Plants, animals, fish, nuts, roots, cereals, grains, eggs and so on.

Tens of thousands of years ago we didn't used to be able to tolerate non-human milk. Now most of us can. We evolve. We change. We adapt. Eat a moderate amount from as much of a wide range as you can and you won't go far wrong.

> ***"Everything in moderation, including moderation."***
> Usually attributed to Oscar Wilde (1854-1900). Playwright and raconteur.

There are however poorer choices and these we can swap for better choices. The principles here are to eat fewer calories and to eat stuff with more fiber. Try to eat less fat but to eat healthier fats if you really must. It's important to eat as much protein as you can manage and to eat stuff which releases its energy more slowly. For a slower energy burn, eat fewer quick release sugars by choosing a slower release complex carbohydrate in its place.

The substitution rules:
- *fewer calories*
- *more fiber*
- *less fat (or healthier)*
- *much more protein*
- *lower GI foods*

Here are my favorites: (I know some of them sound harsh, but I want results - and so do you).

1. Whole milk goes to skimmed fat free. Don't pussy foot around with semi- or 1%. Do it properly.

2. Whole fat yogurt goes to fat-free yogurt. The Greek-style ones are full of flavor.

3. Fruit juice for chilled water with ice cubes and lemon. The same goes for all sodas, carbonated or fizzy drinks. They've got to go. You aren't a child anymore, you need better choices which support your body.

4. White bread and brown bread (yes, brown) swaps to wholegrain and multi-grain versions (soft grain doesn't really count).

5. Swap full fat cheese for lower-fat cheese or cottage cheese.

6. Cheesy sauces with cream get swapped to tomato or roasted vegetable versions.

7. Grill meat, fish and poultry (using the fats already in it) rather than frying. Plus the fats run away and not onto your plate and then into you.

8. Swap muffins and doughnuts for slices of apple, oranges,

raisins and carrot sticks.

9. Cakes and potato chips for rice cakes and lower-fat cream cheese.

10. Swap sugar filled breakfast cereal for whole fruit. Weigh a typical portion for you and then count the calories on the packet - you may be amazed.

11. Instant oatmeal swaps to whole oats. Measure the portions properly. Add skimmed fat-free milk and cook slowly. NO sugar or butter. Heat gently for ten minutes. The grains will still have plenty of roughage and the taste is characteristically nutty. You have calorie control, some protein and a breakfast which will keep you full for hours.

12. Instead of drowning meats in barbecue sauce, cover them in spices and stuff with lemon. The calories are many fewer and because the meat tastes so yummy, you can lose the fatty bits and won't mind that much.

13. Swap mayonnaise for avocado. Mayo is brim full of calories. Avocado has less and you get some vitamins. Consider a half-half mix of avocado and zucchini (courgette). This has even fewer calories, tastes awesome and has lots of fiber (leave the skin on for vitamins, fiber and texture).

14. Ditch ground beef (minced or corned) in favor of grated vegetables. Way more vitamins, fewer calories and some great flavors to boot.

15. Sour cream has fewer calories than plain yogurt. Though not many - but I like the flavor. It's way more interesting.

16. Ditch the croutons on salad. They are carbs deep-fried in oil. Put a few chopped nuts on instead. They taste better and have protein and fiber. Don't go overboard as they are pretty calorific too.

17. Swap roasted, mashed or soup potatoes for cauliflower. It is much better for you, many less unrequired carbohydrates and tastes interesting. A good texture swap and caramelizes to give a lovely smoky flavor. Romanesco looks amazing and can be swapped for the cauliflower. It dry roasts in about ten minutes.

18. Baked potato with butter and cheese swapped to loaded skins with tuna and cottage cheese. Rub the skins with a little salt, bake until crunchy, scoop out most of the low nutritional value soft potato and fill with tuna and a little low-fat soft cheese. Note that sweet potato is crammed full of carbs and nutritionally identical to 'normal' potato, so there is no point in this swap.

19. Swap your fried breakfast for scrambled eggs and smoked salmon. You know why. Yummy and way fewer calories while keeping the high protein content to keep you full until lunchtime.

20. Try cheesecake made in small cups with low fat Greek yogurt and sprinkled with a few fresh berries and a couple of toasted flaked almonds. Dry toast these almonds in a shallow pan until they go lightly brown. Pumpkin seeds do this well too, but better with salt and quite calorific so don't add too many.

21. Swap your latte for an Americano, espresso or macchiato. Much more flavor and you lose the extra calories from the milk.

22. Potato salad with chilled potatoes fills you up much better than French fries and has less fat. And **never** 'go large' - But you don't need me to tell you that!

23. Tandoori chicken has an amazing flavor and the coating has far fewer calories than most curry sauces.

24. Swap cheese, crackers, butter and chutney for cheese and apple slices.

25. Eat a handful of almonds instead of a snack-bar.

26. Frozen yogurt and banana instead of ice cream.

27. A wholegrain wrap has about one hundred calories. Load your sandwich fillings here instead of between two slices of bread at about 120 calories each.

28. Swap milk chocolate for dark chocolate. Fewer calories and you will start to like the taste. Buy the really expensive stuff, it tastes better and you can only afford a smaller quantity.

six
crank up the veg

Eat 4x more
Don't boil them

This point is short: **Eat more veg**. That's it.

If you want to get it right, eat more. Eat more raw.

The protein in vegetables makes them an outstanding eating choice in your quest for a slimmer, trimmer sexier you. The fiber too helps fill you up and keep you fuller for longer.

When we cook food we apply heat to breakdown some of the food structure and alter it chemically. We do this because the flavors change, the textures change and it becomes easier to bite, chew, swallow and digest.

Eating a raw pumpkin takes a long time, but one boiled and mashed goes down nice and easily. When we cook food we break down the naturally occurring fiber. This vital component of vegetables helps our bowels work well, gives us healthy stools and help to stave off bowel cancer. It is good stuff.

Don't destroy your veggies by over-cooking them. You can learn to eat them a little less attacked by the cooking process. As an added bonus they taste better too.

Vegetables are chock full of protein and this is really great for weight loss. It helps us feel full, stay fuller longer and provides vital building blocks for muscles and a healthy life. Vegetables are cheap and can be cooked (or eaten raw) in so very many ways. Eat more.

Eat a lot more. I ask my patients to go away and **quadruple** their intake. I know that they probably won't take me at my word, but at least they start to get the idea.

If you boil veggies, you will leach out the nice vitamin C (*ascorbic acid*) into the water. This is because it is so readily water-soluble. If you then drink the water, no problem. But most of us pour it down the drain. If you steam, grill or roast the veggies you will retain this vital amine.

Roasting vegetables gives them a whole new flavor if you've not tried it before. Try this with their skins on and their skins off as they can taste rather different. Don't overdo it on the oil and fats to roast them in, as these will contain loads of calories you might not want.

Frozen vegetables are excellent. They are cheap, keep in the freezer for years, taste fresh, keep all of their vitamins and are widely available. They cook quickly and can even be microwaved in a couple of minutes (they will usually cook in their own water, so no need to add and then risk losing the lovely vitamin C).

seven
move more each day

Get sweaty
Daily action
Maintain your muscles

Move more. Move a **lot** more. This will help you live longer and happier. Do this while controlling your snack intake and you have the recipe for success.

Moving more builds and maintains muscles. When you see people on hospital wards who are dying, most have fading and puny muscles. Muscles are crucial for a healthy body and need some maintaining. Moving more also builds and maintains fitness. This is combination of how well your heart and lung package work and how efficiently your blood vessels carry the good stuff around and around.

All effective weight loss strategies have the dual aspects of watching intake and increasing daily activities. I didn't say once a week activities. I said **daily**. Really daily. Various government guidelines tell us about the ideal amount of exercise. Often quoted as twenty minutes of vigorous exercise three times a week. That is all well and good but this is a **minimum**. I'll say that again. A minimum to maintain what you've already got. And that includes really old people.

So you and I have fewer excuses. We need to exercise properly several times a week. To keep what you've got. We don't want to keep what we've got. We want to get rid of it. A lot of it. This is going to need a more enthusiastic strategy.

Vigorous exercise should make you sweat. It should make you breathless. Walking doesn't really count. Sex does. I know which I'd rather do. But to keep this up for twenty minutes or more might need a different approach. Swimming, cycling, jogging and running all count. But *only* if you push yourself. You don't need to push yourself to international standard, but to the edge of what you can do. What you can do will increase over time and a few weeks is enough to start noticing real progress.

If you can get these sessions done every day you will make progress. If you can get them done twice a day you will make **much faster progress**. There are some riders; *gradually warm up* over ten minutes of increasing intensity, then *push yourself* so you know you are working hard. Hold that for up to about half an hour. After this do a few minutes *warm down* (such as walking), then do a few minutes of *stretching*. Do the stretches on warm muscles (swinging your limbs wildly with cold muscles makes it more likely you will sprain a muscle or two).

Your muscles will adapt. All of them. Your biceps, your thighs, your abs, your glutes. The muscles that keep your core posture, your pelvis floor and the muscles that raise your eyebrows. If you do more with these muscles they will grow, if you do less they will shrink.

For a healthy body you will need to work your body and use it each and every day. Do this with plenty of protein in your diet and everything else will just work better (your brain, your sleep, your immune system and your cancer repairing system). Plus your sex drive and enjoyment of sex will improve. Most of us like that bit.

eight
sleep better

Eight hours each night
Avoid wees
Evening deliberately dehydrate
Morning bright light to set the system
Why?
Mental sorting
Avoid sedatives

You will be thinner if you sleep better and you will be fatter if you skimp on vital shut-eye.

A bold claim, to be sure. But true. People find it hard to lose weight if their head doesn't feel good. The number one cause of your head not being up to scratch is lack of sleep. Handily it is one of the easiest things to fix and get right.

We all need about eight hours a night. But we get on average six to seven hours. We go to bed late because we watch TV and go out in the evenings. We answer emails, surf the web, check our social media sites, text and catch up with Twitter. We then take ages to get off to sleep, are rudely wakened by the alarm clock and use caffeine to power us through the next day. At the weekend we stay up even later but treat ourselves to lie-ins in an attempt to catch up a bit.

We are usually too tired during the weekend to get some serious exercise in. Each year it's getting worse. Nearly all of my patients in my weight clinic don't get good sleep. When you put on weight, you also find it harder to sleep. Fat accumulates under our chins causing breathing impairment by night and leading to light, interrupted, non-restorative sleep (as well as a potentially fatal heart condition).

Being sleep deprived leads to increased death from car accidents, depression, suicide and increased heart disease. It probably also increases your risk of serious infections and cancer. As if that weren't bad enough, it also makes you more likely to binge eat, binge drink and make poor food choices throughout the day - particularly the evening.

If this doesn't apply to you, well done. But you are in the minority. The rest of us struggle.

So what to do? Good question. The answers are as follows, do them and everything else will get better:

1. Make sleep a priority. Not something you will squeeze in.
2. Go to bed early. No more than one late night a week, plan it and make it special if you like.
3. Get a pre-sleep routine (teeth, face, pajamas, read quietly, light off).
4. Get up at the same time each day. Your body-clock likes this.
5. Sleep in a dark room. Use black-out blinds if needed.
6. Sleep with no noise interruptions. Use a white noise if you need (there are lots of ten hour free videos on the interweb).
7. Try not to urinate at night. If you do, fluid restrict yourself the previous evening. If you still do, speak to your doctor.
8. Avoid caffeine. Avow to avoid all caffeine for a few weeks until you are settled, then none after midday (as it stays in your system for many hours, is cumulative and stops you getting off well).
9. Keep a dream diary, wake up and write them down. This will become easier with time and dreaming well decreases anxiety and depression.
10. Keep a worry diary. Write down three things on your mind before you go to bed. This will help your unconscious brain sort through this while you sleep, which decreases stress levels.

11. Keep a grateful diary. Think of three things you are grateful for each night as you drift off to sleep. This promotes better rest.

12. Avoid all sedatives, these stop your frontal lobes from sorting through information from the day, creating memories and increasing your intelligence. Don't forget, alcohol is a sedative.

13. Get bright light each morning, it helps reset your body clock. Go outside for a walk.

14. Avoid bright light in the two hours before your bed-time. This particularly includes the blue spectrum light from TV, all electronic devices and computer screens. Real books and e-readers are far superior here.

15. Don't forget your daily bout of exercise (and yes, it *can* be in the evening, as crazy as that might sound having read this list).

nine
be busy

When you exercise you don't eat (double whammy of bonuses)
Distract yourself
Get focused on a project

If you are doing something that requires your whole concentration, you will tend to snack less. If you are running away from a sabre-toothed tiger or romping with the bed-partner(s) of your dreams, you might not think about food until you are done. As a benefit, what you are doing will be burning calories for double bonus points.

The more time during the day you are busy, the better you will do on your better-waistline mission. Do this deliberately. Plan ahead.

Your willpower is a limited resource, just like a phone battery. It charges up overnight and with proper rest (and I mean eight or more hours here). Each time you resist a temptation, it will fade a little. Eventually you will struggle with these temptations. We all will, it is human nature and not a weakness of your character or soul.

"I can resist anything but temptation."
Oscar Wilde. Lady Windermere's Fan, 1892, Act I

The trick is to realize this will happen and plan around it. If you use it as an excuse, then you will stay the same shape as you are today.

Plan ahead and keep no snacks to hand when you are being busy on a project. When you are doing something, focus on this alone and turn off all distractions. There are **no** tweets, instant messages, emails, news updates or new videos of funny cats which won't wait for an hour of your life. Nothing you do is THAT important. Really. Close the screens down, hide the pop-up message and banner alerts, turn off the sounds and vibrates. Do one thing, the thing in front of you, until the top of the hour ticks by - set an alarm for that if you like. Then spend five or ten minutes or whatever you choose and answer all that stuff. Turn it all off again and continue.

Do this throughout the day and you will get way more done, you will feel better and you will not be sapping your concentration or willpower.

I suggest phone calls are included. Have your voicemail on and go through everything after that hour mark. We are all guilty of it. But you wouldn't want a surgeon who was operating on you to be checking text messages and you wouldn't expect a pilot flying your plane to glance through what is happening on their Twitter feed. Is your job and what you are doing so rubbish that you have different standards for other people? No, I thought not. Do what you are doing, do it well and then get to your social and other business life.

Try it today, do it for a week and I challenge you not to find it changes your life to the good. For good. It will feel weird at first, that's normal. All new habits take a good few weeks to groove and during this time they take a bit of effort. That gradually fades until they are automatic. You will manage more than any of your colleagues. Less than half a per cent of working adults do this. What an easy way to get a competitive edge.

And you'll eat less.

ten
work on mood

Learn to just say no
Ask for help
Don't be a victim

They say that all good things come to those who wait. I reckon
that sloth, arthritis and an early grave would phrase it better. In
my experience and probably yours too: All good things come to
those who work jolly hard at it day after day. And *then* you need
a hefty dose of luck and good genes to begin with.

Mental health and wellbeing is no exception. No one talks
much about mental health which is a shame as it is REALLY
important. If your head isn't in the right place you can eat as
many rice crackers as you like, but you are still going to binge
on snacks when you are a bit lonely and sad.

I exaggerate. But only a little. The patients who do badly are
usually those whose mental happiness isn't what it could or
should be. Not really rocket science, but worth mentioning.

Your mood is the single biggest thing in the way of you being
the right shape.

Really.

If I am grumpy, tired, angry, lonely, stressed, bored or lusty I
don't think straight. Nor do you. Nor does anyone. It's normal
but not really ok. If your head is not straight, you won't look
after your body well, will tend to eat junk, will not sleep well
and you are not likely to get enough decent (or indecent)
exercise.

Sort this out before anything else. I agree it isn't always easy. If
it was, it wouldn't be a problem. But ignore this at your peril.

Until you can iron out these wrinkles in your life, the mission for a hot, sexy body just isn't going to work out well for you.

Treat your head-state as your number one priority and everything else will start to fall into place. If it doesn't I will refund you the price of this book. And possibly eat my hat too.

Being in the best mood you can be will make a huge difference to your day. The key to this is taking action in not playing the part of a victim. Don't be a victim of your circumstances. Sure you will be busy, the kids will bother you, your mother will come to stay, the milk will spill and you will forget to pay a bill. The weather will be too hot, too cold, too wet, too whatever. The point is that all our lives are busy. Some have it lucky. Some don't. We will have good days and bad.

When the luck of the day had dealt you a rubbish hand you will not get any stuff done if you feel sorry for yourself. Shrug it off, get over it and do something about it. Your mood will improve if you decide to. Simply decide to be ok with whatever is happening in your life. Change the stuff you can and put everything else in a mental box. Leave all that for another day.

If you need help with that, then go and get some. Don't be a victim of your life circumstances. They may be terrible. I know, we all have awful stuff happen. Sometimes it's not that bad. In ten years time, a lot of it won't seem quite so terrible (though some will). But you have things to get done, you need to do stuff. You need to focus and pay attention to making your life healthy with a smaller waistline. You need to do this today. To get on track with your current mission to shape up, you will need to focus on the here and now. Start with a smile and affect the things you can. If it doesn't feel like you are on a fabulous crusade to improve your life and wellbeing, then stop reading. Go back to the start because you've probably missed something.

common derailers 1
can't get started

Start small
Start huge
Need a bigger goal
Need a better motivator

Stuff that stops us just as soon as we get started is a pain in the rear end. We don't want it but can't get away from it. If these things happen to you, smile, pat yourself on the back for noticing, dust yourself off and start again.

If you can't get started there are four things to get your head around; start small, start huge, get a bigger goal, get better motivation.

To **start small**, try sneaking up on yourself. This is the human, modern, clever part of your brain fooling the powerful but stupid animal brain. You can sneak up on it by doing lots of tiny things it can't object to. Walk ten extra steps a day. Leave one forkful at each meal. Pile less on your plate to leave it a tiny bit less full. Do these, do them each day and then increase them step by step. Within a few weeks, the difference will be noticeable.

Another way to get started is to **make a massive commitment**. Something so massive that you have no choice but to rearrange your life around it just to fit it in. An all or nothing thing. Enter a marathon, commit to losing forty pounds, bet your house on reaching a certain sized waistline. That sort of thing. You will find something you are comfortable with, but it works better if you feel the pressure. Then you will have to do stuff each and every day to achieve it. You can't afford off days. You won't be able to afford to let the ball slip. I like this method. I know it's not for everyone, but if you've got the *chutzpah* to try it, the results can be life-changing.

If you aren't doing the stuff you need to do each day to support your goal, perhaps your goal isn't big enough. It doesn't inspire you or motivate you enough. Go back and rethink your goal. Rewrite it. Why are you doing this? Why bother to read this? Why bother to try and change your life for the better?

Do you want to stay as you are? Ok, why not? What do you want instead? Ask yourself these questions, write down your answers and check back in with them when you meet a low point. If they don't motivate you then, that's the time to go back and re-do them. You can re-write your goals and change them as often as you like. That's ok, and even encouraged if they aren't getting you off your butt and into action. Go on, what are you waiting for?

common derailers 2
fell off wagon

Strategy
Will happen
How will you manage?

When you fall off the wagon, you will need a plan. You might not and pigs might fly. The question is how long will you be off for before you a) notice and b) do something constructive about it. Beating yourself up for being a weak person will not help. Stop that. Find something else. Check in with your goals, phone a friend, go for a walk, run around the block, have a massage. Don't eat chocolate and cookies, that is not the right place for comfort. Have a plan. Maybe write that plan down right next to your goals and go to this piece of paper when trouble strikes (keep the piece of paper somewhere you can always find it, like your undies drawer). Stuff crops up. Life is like that. If you plan ahead, this can make a huge difference. You could even re-read this book!

common derailers 3
no progress

Not doing enough
Balance
Be negative
Bigger effort
Sustain for longer
More realistic

If you are still flatlining with your progress then thinking about the energy balance has to come next. Most of us, I was going to say my patients, but I do too, underestimate the calories we put in and overestimate how much exercise we really do. The **three** quick fixes are to **do some exercise each day** (sometimes we let this slip), **decrease our portion sizes** (smaller plates and obsessively weighing everything are the fastest fixers) and **make sure we're getting enough sleep** (that one tends to slide when we are up against it in our lives and need to do more. But to do more, we need to do less… at night. The saw cuts better when it is sharp).

common derailers 4
end of the day

Small failures can add up to a lot
Watch for hoovering calories at low points

When you fall off the wagon, that is ok. It is normal and may even happen every day. Possibly more than once a day on bad days. But it is what you do about it which will determine your results. If you can notice, then readjust without delay, you will do amazing things. Great stuff awaits you.

The last thing to say is a warning about how most of us fall off the wagon. Every day. We hoover up the calories at low points. Physical low points. Mental, psychological, emotional or spiritual low points are just as bad. When you feel like this, the warning signs are there. This should ring a big fat alarm bell. Watch out for this. Notice it. Spot this early, try to head these situations off from happening. Don't have snacks to hand. Have no food in your drawer, purse or car. Eat little and often. Eat healthy stuff in advance, don't get tired. Get help early for all the things in your life which pressure you. Find stuff you enjoy and which recharges your batteries. Go and do this often.

I wish you the best of luck. And when luck doesn't work, stop, take a big breath, ask for help and have another go.

summary pointers

Check-in checklist

- Weight loss is straightforward, though not always easy.

- It has to matter enough to you.

- Consistency is key.

- If you fall off, pick yourself up, dust yourself off and get on with it again.

- Do stuff which helps.

- Small things each and every day.

- Get better day on day, week on week.

- Help someone else. This can unlock the secrets in your mind as you become focused on the task at hand and then have the social pressure to be the best you can be.

about the author

I hope you enjoyed this book and find that it really helps. I'd love you to leave a review online.

Dr Phil Harley is a family practitioner in the UK. For twenty years he has helped people get into the best shape they can be as a GP and weight loss expert. In his spare time he enjoys running ultramarathons. Rather slowly.

Let me know how it goes. Let me know about your goals and when you reach your targets. Show off. Get to feel smug. Drop me an email. If you have any questions, feedback or suggestions. Please get in touch at drphil@brainsolutions.co.uk

For more books by Dr Harley check out www.brainsolutions.co.uk

Also available:

Skinny Genes - *Weight Gain Explained & the CURE*

Desert Marathon Training - *2nd edition*

Beginner's Guide to Running

Ultramarathon Running Injuries - *Niggles, Scrapes and Nipple Chafes*

30 Winning Weight Loss Ways - *Simple, easy, step-by-step expert diet guidance*

Coming soon:

Do it, Do it, *DO IT!* - *A Procrastinator's Guide to World Domination*

Stand Up Sexy - *Perfect Posture for Everyday & Better Bedroom Fun. Cure Back Pain - A Doctor's Guide*

BetterDay - *Do Stuff Better. Today*

www.ingramcontent.com/pod-product-compliance
Lightning Source LLC
Chambersburg PA
CBHW070339190526
45169CB00005B/1960